50+ Plant-Based Diet Dessert Ideas

Simple and Yummy Dessert Collection

Luke Gorman

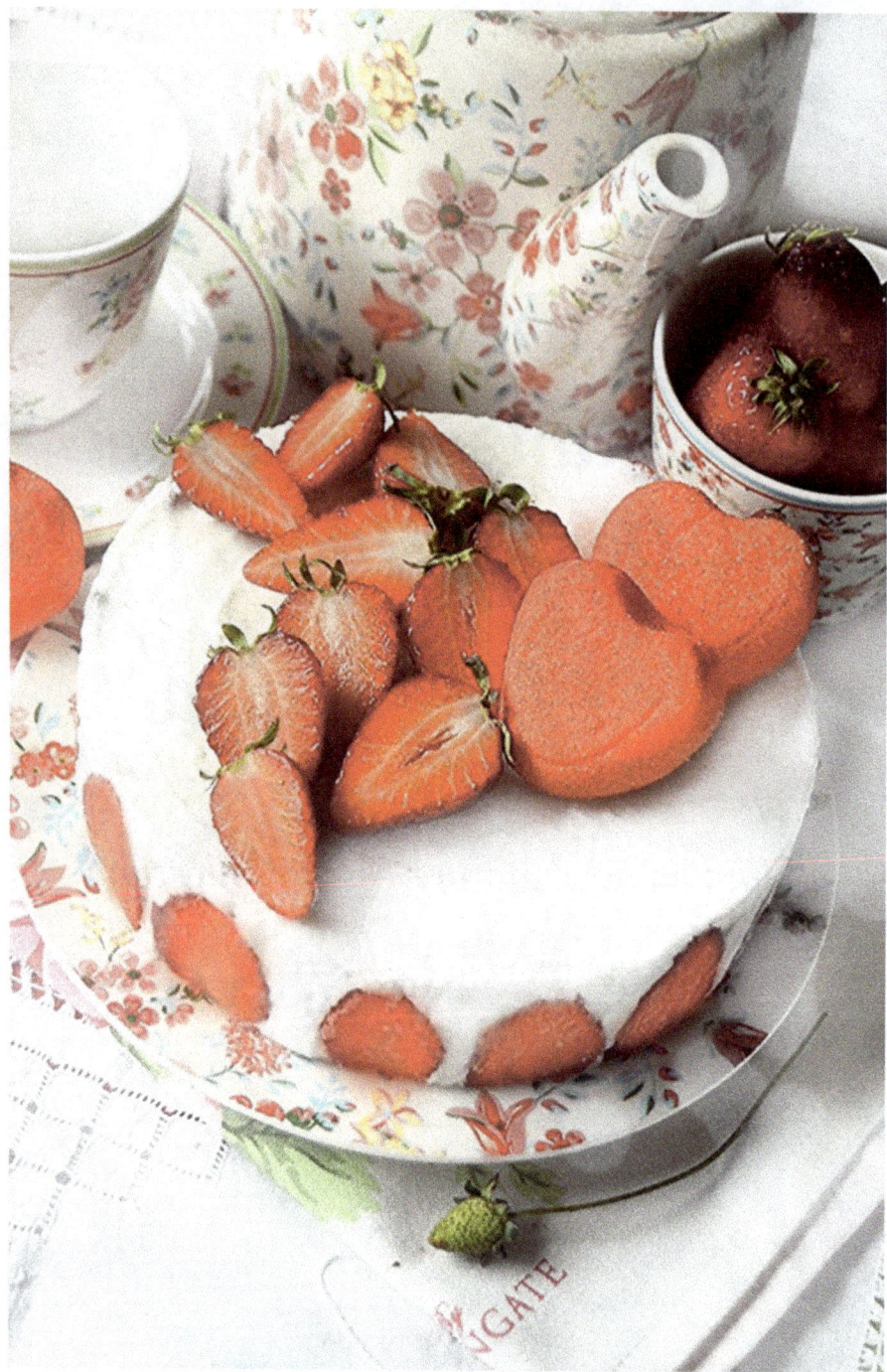

TABLE OF CONTENTS

Introduction

A plant-based eating routine backing and upgrades the entirety of this. For what reason should most of what we eat originate from the beginning?

Eating more plants is the first nourishing convention known to man to counteract and even turn around the ceaseless diseases that assault our general public.

Plants and vegetables are brimming with large scale and micronutrients that give our bodies all that we require for a sound and productive life. By eating, at any rate, two suppers stuffed with veggies consistently, and nibbling on foods grown from the ground in the middle of, the nature of your wellbeing and at last your life will improve.

The most widely recognized wellbeing worries that individuals have can be reduced by this one straightforward advance.

Things like weight, inadequate rest, awful skin, quickened maturing, irritation, physical torment, and absence of vitality would all be able to be decidedly influenced by expanding the admission of plants and characteristic nourishments.

If you're reading this book, then you're probably on a journey to get healthy because you know good health and nutrition go hand in hand.

Maybe you're looking at the plant-based diet as a solution to those love handles.

Whatever the case may be, the standard American diet millions of people eat daily is not the best way to fuel your body.

If you ask me, any other diet will already be a significant improvement. Since what you eat fuels your body, you can imagine that eating junk will make you feel just that—like junk.

I've followed the standard American diet for several years: my plate was loaded with high-fat and carbohydrate-rich foods. I know this doesn't sound like a horrible way to eat, but keep in mind that most Americans don't focus on eating healthy fats and complex carbs—we live on processed foods.

The consequences of eating foods filled with trans fats, preservatives, and mountains of sugar are fatigue, reduced mental focus, mood swings, and weight gain. To top it off, there's the issue of opening yourself up to certain diseases—some life-threatening—when you neglect paying attention to what you eat .

Vegan Lemon Meringue Pie

Preparation time: 15 minutes

Cooking time: 45 minutes 8 slices.

Ingredients:

- 1 ½ cups sugar

- 1/3 up cornstarch

- ½ tsp. salt

- ½ tsp. agar

- 1 cup water

- 1 ½ cup coconut milk

- 2 tbsp. lemon zest

- 1 cup lemon juice

Meringue Ingredients:

10 tbsp. egg replacer

5 tbsp. chilled water

1 ¼ cup sugar

1 prepared pie crust (store bought)

Lemon Pie

Directions:

1. Begin by adding the first group of ingredients: from the sugar to the lemon juice, to the saucepan.

2. Allow the mixture to boil, stirring all the time.

3. After it becomes very thick, pour the mixture into the pie pan.

4. Next, preheat the oven to 210 degrees Fahrenheit.

5. In a separate bowl, mix together the egg replacer with the chilled water.

6. Stir well, creating soft white peaks.

7. Now, add the sugar.

8. Mix slowly so that the meringue is super-thick and will refuse to fall down if tipped over.

9. Next, scoop this meringue over the chilled lemon filling, prepared above, and then allow the pie to sit for twenty minutes.

10. Now, allow the pie to cook in the oven for thirty minutes.

11. Allow the pie to cool after baking, and serve.

12. Enjoy.

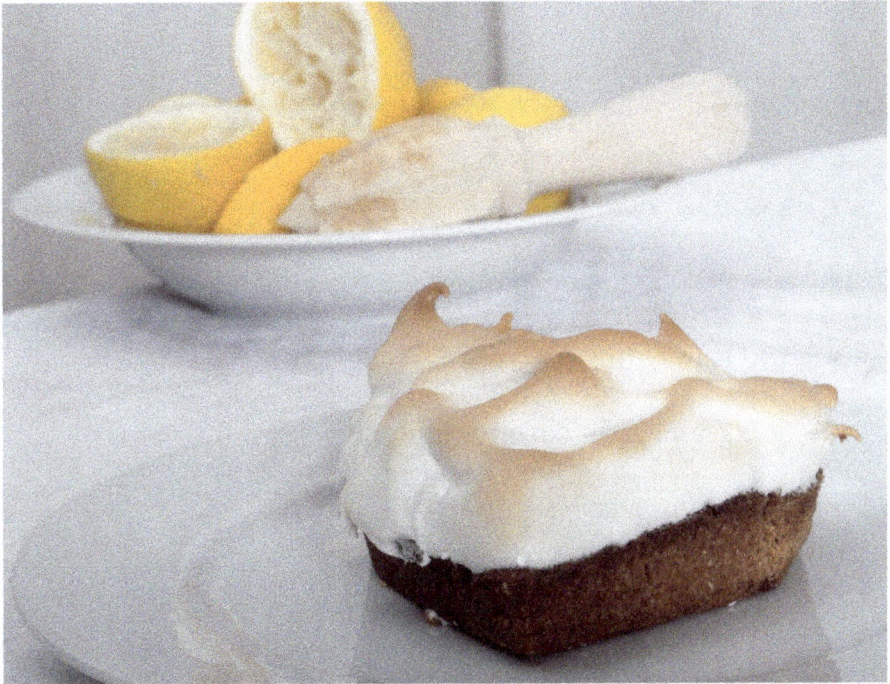

Vegan Vanilla Ice Cream

Preparation time: 15 minutes

Cooking time: 45 minutes

2 cups.

Ingredients:

- 3 vanilla pods
- 1 ½ tsp. vanilla bean paste
- 400 ml soymilk
- 600 grams light coconut milk
- 200 grams agave syrup

Directions:

1. Begin by slicing the vanilla pods and removing the seeds.

2. Place the seeds in a big mixing bowl and toss out the pods.

3. Next, add the rest of the ingredients, and position the ingredients into an ice cream maker.

4. Churn the ice cream for forty-five minutes.

5. Next, place the mixture into a freezer container, and allow the ice cream to freeze for three hours.

6. Serve, and enjoy!

Vegan Cupcakes

Preparation time: 15 minutes

Cooking time: 55 minutes

Servings: 5

Ingredients:

- 1 ¼ tsp vanilla extract

- ½ tsp salt

- 2 tsp baking soda

- 5 tbsp. Splenda

- 1 ½ cups almond milk

- ½ cup coconut oil, warmed until liquid

- ½ tsp baking powder

- 2 cups almond flour

- 1 tbsp apple cider vinegar

Directions:

1. Set the oven at 350 degrees.

2. Spread oil or butter on 12 muffin tins.

3. You can also cover it with paper liners if desired.

4. Pour the apple cider in a cup.

5. Add enough almond milk to make it 1 ½ cups.

6. Set it aside for 5 minutes until it curdles.

7. Whisk the flour, baking powder, salt, sugar and baking soda.

8. Pour the mixture to the dry mixture and whisk to combine.

9. Scoop the batter into the muffin tins.

10. Bake for 15-20 minutes until it is done.

11. Remove from the oven and let it cool in a wire rack.

12. Arrange in a platter and decorate it as desired.

Lemon Bars

Preparation time: 15 minutes

Cooking time: 25 minutes

Servings: 5

Ingredients:

- 3/4 cup melted butter

- 3/4 cup almond flour

- 1 1/2 cups boiling water

- 2/3 cup lemon gelatin mix, no sugar added

- 3 Tbsp freshly squeezed lemon juice

- 12 oz cream cheese

Directions:

1. Set the oven to 350 degrees F.

2. Combine the melted butter and flour together in a bowl, then pour the mixture into a baking pan, pressing down to create a crust.

3. Bake for 10 minutes then set on a cooling rack.

4. Cool completely before use.

5. In a large mixing bowl, mix the gelatin and boiling water.

6. Stir until the gelatin completely dissolves.

7. Stir in the lemon juice and cream cheese, mixing well.

8. Pour the mixture on top of the crust, then place in the refrigerator and chill overnight, or for 3 hours at least.

9. Slice into 12 servings.

Chocolate Peanut Butter Smoothie

Preparation time: 30 minutes

Cooking time: 0 minutes

Servings: 01

Ingredients:

- 1 cup almond milk

- ¼ cup quick oats

- 1 scoop plant-based protein powder

- 2 tablespoons peanut butter

- 2 teaspoons cocoa powder

- 1 tablespoon maple syrup

- 1 cup ice

Directions:

1. Add all ingredients to a blender.

2. Hit the pulse button and blend till it is smooth.

3. Chill well to serve.

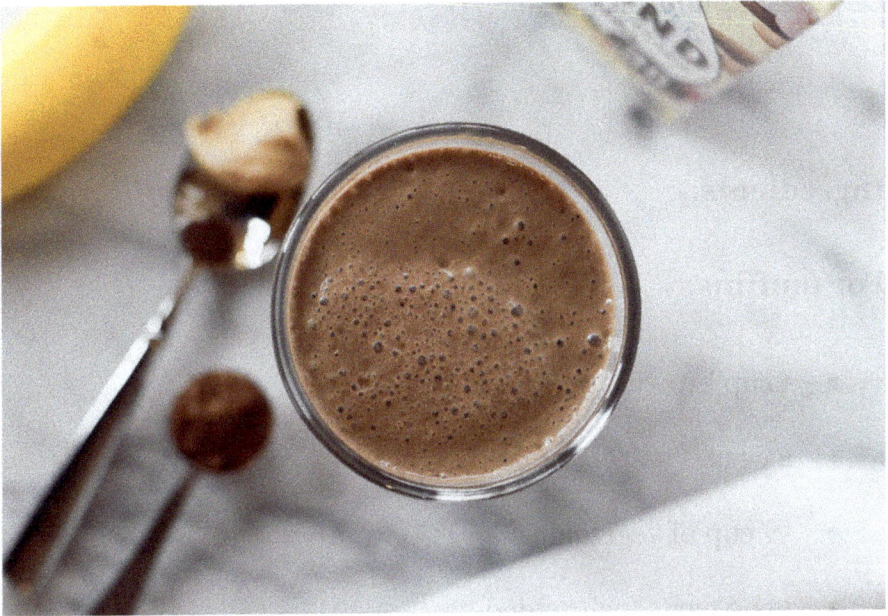

Carrot cake muffins

Preparation time: 10 minutes

Cooking time: 20 minutes

Servings: 12 muffins

Ingredients:

For muffins:

- 1 cup brown sugar

- 2 eggs

- ½ cup of vegetable oil

- 1 cup carrots shredded

- ½ cup milk

- 1 ½ cup flour

- 1 tsp baking powder

- 1 tsp baking soda

- 1 tsp cinnamon

- ¼ tsp salt

Frosting:

- ¼ cup butter
- ¼ cup cream cheese
- 2 ½ cup icing sugar
- ¼ tsp vanilla
- Salt a pinch
- 2tbsp Cream

Directions:

1. Preheat oven at 400 degrees.
2. Set the muffin pan with oil grease and flour dust.
3. Take a medium bowl and whisk vegetable oil, eggs, carrot, and milk.
4. In another bowl, mix the dry Ingredients like sugar, flour, baking powder, baking soda, cinnamon and salt.
5. Now mix the dry Ingredients into the batter with the help of spatula until smooth.

6. Now pour the batter into a muffin pan and bake it for 20 minutes.

7. Prepare the cream frosting in a bowl by adding the butter, icing sugar, cream cheese, cream, salt and vanilla extract, beat them until frothy.

8. Serve the muffin with the cream cheese frosting.

Peanut butter stuffed dates

Preparation time: 5 minutes

Cooking time: 5 minutes

Servings: 6

Ingredients:

- 6 medjool dates
- 6tsp peanut butter
- Chocolate crunches or coconut for topping

Directions:

1. Take 6 dates, wash them and let them dry.
2. Now remove the pits from the dates without splitting them into half.
3. Fill each date with a tablespoon of peanut butter.
4. Set them in the refrigerator to get cold for a while.
5. Now cut the dates from the center half.
6. Top each with different topping and serve chilled.

Trouble Chocolate-Chocolate Cookies

Preparation time: 15 minutes

Cooking time: 25 minutes

12 cookies.

Ingredients:

- 1 tsp. vanilla

- ½ cup cane sugar

- 1/3 cup brown sugar

- 1/3 cup sunflower seed butter

- 1/3 cup coconut oil

- 1 tbsp. ground flax

- 3 tbsp. water

- 2 cups oats (processed in food processor)

- 2 tsp. soymilk

- ½ tsp. baking powder

- ½ tsp. baking soda

- 1 chopped nondairy chocolate bar

Directions:

1. Begin by preheating the oven to 350 degrees Fahrenheit.

2. Next, mix together the flax and the water in a big mixing bowl.

3. Set this to the side for five minutes.

4. Next, add all of the first five ingredients to the flax seed bowl and stir well.

5. Next, add the dry ingredients to the bowl.

6. Stir well between each addition.

7. Add the soymilk last to moisten the dough.

8. Chop up the chocolate and add the chocolate to the batter, stirring quickly.

9. Create dough balls and place the dough balls on a baking sheet.

10. Press at them a bit, and bake them for thirteen minutes.

11. Cool them for about fifteen minutes, and enjoy!

Miami Mango Shake

Preparation time: 30 minutes

Cooking time: 0 minutes

Servings: 01

Ingredients:

- 1 cup unsweetened coconut milk

- 1 scoop protein powder

- 1 cup frozen mango

- 1 cup frozen strawberries

Directions:

1. Add all ingredients to a blender.

2. Hit the pulse button and blend till it is smooth.

3. Chill well to serve.

Iced Tea

Preparation time: 5 minutes

Cooking time: 0 minutes

Servings: 2

Ingredients:

- A cup high quality tea bag

- A tablespoon of coconut butter

- A tablespoon of plant-based milk of your choice

Optional add-ins:

- 1 teaspoon of MCT oil

- 1 teaspoon of cinnamon

- 1 teaspoon of vanilla powder

- 1 teaspoon of coconut milk powder (instead of the plant milk)

Directions:

1. Brew your coffee – either a French press or automatic coffee maker using high-quality coffee.

2. Add a cup of coffee in a blender along with coconut butter and other add-ins and blend until foamy.

3. Pour in a mug and top with foamed plant milk or dust with cinnamon.

Strawberry-Choco Shake

Preparation time: 5 minutes

Cooking time: 0 minutes

Servings: 1

Ingredients:

- ½ cup heavy cream, liquid

- 1 tbsp cocoa powder

- 1 packet Stevia, or more to taste

- 4 strawberries, sliced

- 1 tbsp coconut flakes, unsweetened

What you'll need from the store cupboard:

- 1 ½ cups water

- 3 tbsps coconut oil

Directions

1. Add all ingredients in a blender.

2. Blend until smooth and creamy.

3. Serve and enjoy.

Creamy Choco Shake

Preparation time: 5 minutes

Cooking time: 0 minutes

Servings: 1

Ingredients:

- ½ cup heavy cream
- 2 tbsp cocoa powder
- 1 packet Stevia, or more to taste
- 1 cup water

What you'll need from the store cupboard:

- 3 tbsps coconut oil

Directions

1. Add all ingredients in a blender.
2. Blend until smooth and creamy.
3. Serve and enjoy.

No Cook Coconut and Chocolate Bars

Preparation time: 15 minutes

Cooking time: 0 minutes

Servings: 6

Ingredients:

- 1 tbsp Stevia

- ¾ cup shredded coconut, unsweetened

- ½ cup ground nuts (almonds, pecans, or walnuts)

- ¼ cup unsweetened cocoa powder

- 4 tbsp coconut oil

What you'll need from the store cupboard:

1. Done

Directions

2. In a medium bowl, mix shredded coconut, nuts, and cocoa powder.

3. Add Stevia and coconut oil.

4. Mix batter thoroughly.

5. In a 9x9 square inch pan or dish, press the batter and for a 30-minutes place in the freezer.

6. Serve and enjoy.

Chocolate Mousse

Preparation time: 15 minutes

Cooking time: 0 minutes

Servings: 4

Ingredients:

- 1 large, ripe avocado

- 1/4 cup sweetened almond milk

- 1 tbsp coconut oil

- ¼ cup cocoa or cacao powder

- 1 tsp vanilla extract

What you'll need from the store cupboard:

- none

Directions

1. In a food processor, process all ingredients until smooth and creamy.

2. Transfer to a lidded container and chill for at least 4 hours.

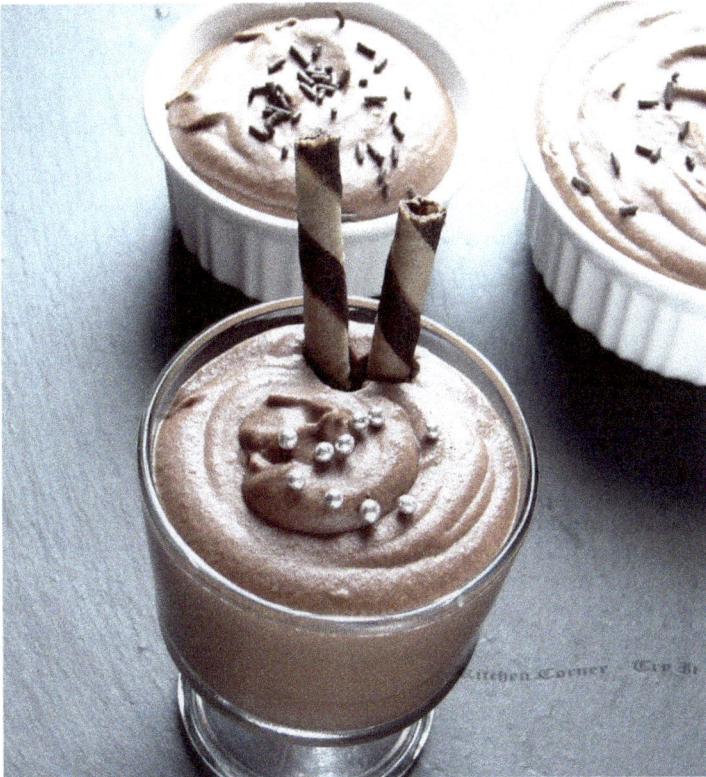

3. Serve and enjoy.

Apple Tart

Preparation time: 5 minutes

Cooking time: 40 minutes

Servings: 4

Ingredients:

crust

- 1 ⅓ cups flour

- ¼ tsp. salt

- 1 Tbs. sugar

- ½ cup butter, well chilled scant

- ⅓ cup ice water filling

- 2 lbs. firm pippin apples

- juice of 1 large lemon

- ½ cup sugar

- ½ to ⅓ cup apricot glaze (optional)

Directions:

1. To make the crust, mix together the flour, salt, and 1 tablespoon of sugar, then cut in the butter with a pastry blender or two sharp knives until the mixture resembles coarse corn meal.

2. Sprinkle the ice water over it and toss together quickly until the flour is evenly moistened and the dough is starting to hold together.

3. Form the dough into a ball and chill it for 1 hour, then roll it out in a 12-inch circle and fit it into a 10½-inch false-bottom quiche tin or flan ring.

4. Trim off the excess, leaving a ¼-inch rim above the pan, and flute the rim with the blunt edge of a butter knife.

5. Chill the shell for ½ hour.

6. Line the shell with foil and fill it with dried beans or rice.

7. Bake in a preheated oven at 425 degrees for 8 minutes, then remove the beans and foil, prick the shell in several places with a fork, and put it back in the oven for 4 to 5 minutes, just until the bottom of the crust begins to color.

8. Meanwhile, peel and core the apples and cut them in even, lengthwise slices, no thicker than ¼ inch at the outside.

9. Put the apple slices in a bowl with the lemon juice and ½ cup of the sugar, toss lightly, and leave them there for 45 minutes.

10. Drain the apples and reserve the liquid.

11. The partially baked crust can be painted with apricot glaze before the apples are arranged on it.

12. This is one more way to fight the soggy crust problem.

13. Heat up the glaze and brush it on lightly with a pastry brush.

14. Arrange the apple slices neatly in the crust by very closely overlapping them in concentric circles, starting at the outside edge.

15. Use all the apples.

16. Sprinkle the remaining sugar (about 3 tablespoons) evenly over the apples.

17. Bake the tart for 30 to 35 minutes in a preheated oven at 375 degrees.

18. The apples should just be starting to brown at the edges.

19. While the tart is baking, boil the reserved liquid from the apples until it is reduced to a medium-thick, glazelike consistency.

20. When the tart is done, brush the apples lightly with this glaze, or drizzle it over them.

21. Serve the tart warm or cool, with or without the apricot glaze.

Lemon Torte

Preparation time: 5 minutes

Cooking time: 40 minutes

Servings: 2

Ingredients:

- 1¼ cups egg whites

- 2 cups confectioners' sugar

- 2 Tbs. cornstarch

- ¼ tsp. almond extract

- 1 ⅔ cups ground almonds (unblanched)

- Lemon Filling blanched almond halves

Directions:

1. Beat the egg whites with 1 cup of the confectioners' sugar until they hold soft peaks.

2. Sift together the second cup of sugar and the cornstarch, add it to the egg whites along with the almond extract, and continue beating until the egg whites are stiff.

3. Fold in the ground almonds. Butter and flour two 10-inch cake pans and divide the beaten egg white mixture between them, spreading it as flat and smooth as possible.

4. Bake the layers in a preheated oven at 275 degrees for 1½ hours.

5. They should be pale gold in color and shrinking away from the sides of the pan.

6. Allow the layers to cool slightly in the pans, then carefully remove them and let them finish cooling on racks.

7. Spread a little more than half the lemon filling on one layer and place the second layer on top of it.

8. Spread the remaining filling over the top and sides of the top layer, leaving the sides of the bottom layer exposed.

9. Decorate the torte very simply with a few blanched almond halves or just swirl the lemon topping evenly with a butter knife and leave it plain.

10. Chill the torte for at least an hour.

Nuts Balls

Preparation time: 10 minutes

Cooking time: 20 minutes

Servings: 12

Ingredients:

- 2 tablespoons flaxseed mixed with 3 tablespoons water
- 1 cup almonds, chopped
- 1 cup macadamia nuts, chopped
- ½ cup walnuts, chopped
- 1 cup coconut cream
- ¼ cup coconut, unsweetened and shredded
- ½ cup cashew cheese, grated
- Salt and black pepper to the taste
- 1 tablespoon Italian seasoning
- 2 tablespoons coconut oil, melted

- Cooking spray

Directions:

1. In a bowl, combine the flaxseed with the nuts, cream and the other ingredients except the cooking spray, whisk well and shape medium balls out of the mix.
2. Arrange the balls on a baking sheet lined with parchment paper, grease with cooking spray and bake at 400 degrees F for 20 minutes.
3. Arrange the balls on a platter and serve.

Kale & Avocado Smoothie

Preparation Time: 10 minutes

Cooking Time: 0 minute

Servings: 1

Ingredients:

- 1 ripe banana

- 1 cup kale

- 1 cup almond milk

- ¼ avocado

- 1 tbsp. chia seeds

- 2 tsp. honey

- 1 cup ice cubes

Direction:

1. Blend all the ingredients until smooth.

Orange & Carrot Juice

Preparation Time: 15 minutes

Cooking Time: 0 minute

Servings: 2

Ingredients:

- 1 tomato, sliced
- 1 orange, sliced into wedges
- 1 apple, sliced
- 4 carrots, sliced
- Ice cubes

Direction:

1. Follow the order of the ingredients list when processing these through the juice.
2. Transfer the juice into glasses.
3. Fill your glass with ice and serve.

Sweet and Hot Nuts

Preparation time: 5 minutes

Cooking time: 4 hours;

Servings: 12

Ingredients:

- ½ pound assorted nuts, raw

- 1/3 cup butter, melted

- 1 teaspoon cayenne pepper or to taste

- 1 tablespoon MCT oil or coconut oil

What you'll need from the store cupboard:

- 1 packet stevia powder

- ¼ tsp salt

Directions

1. Place all ingredients in the crockpot.

2. Give it a good stir to combine everything.

3. Close the lid and cook on low for 4 hours.

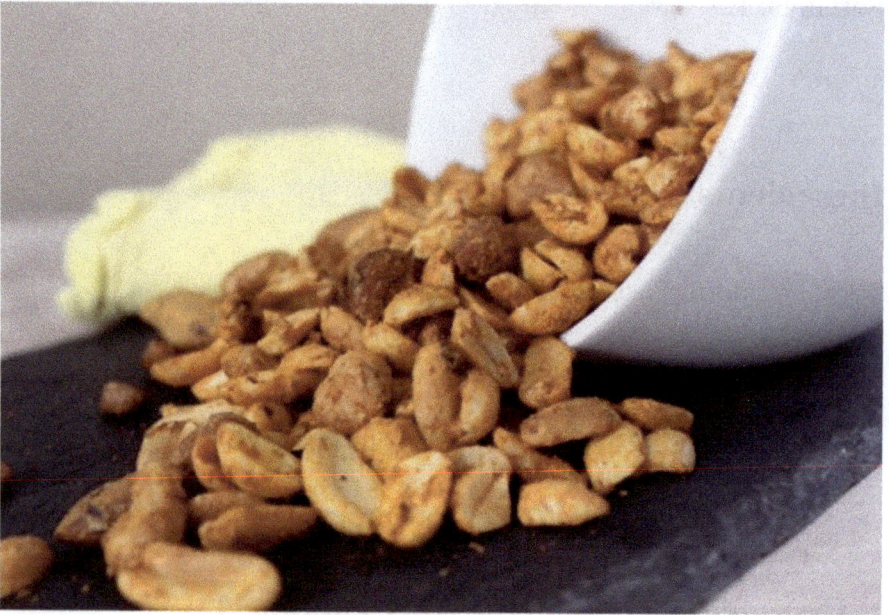

Sponge Cake

Preparation time: 5 minutes

Cooking time: 20 minutes

Servings: 4

Ingredients:

- 6 eggs, separated
- 1 cup sugar
- ¼ cup boiling water
- 1 Tbs. lemon juice
- ½ tsp. vanilla extract
- 1½ cups flour
- 1½ tsp. baking powder
- pinch of salt
- 4 Tbs. olive oil

Directions:

1. Beat the egg yolks until they are creamy and light, then gradually add the sugar a bit at a time, while you continue beating.

2. Beat the yolks and sugar together until the mixture is pale colored and fluffy—another 10 minutes or so.

3. Gradually add the boiling water, lemon juice, and vanilla and beat another few minutes.

4. Sift together the flour and baking powder and fold it into the egg yolk mixture.

5. Beat the egg whites with a pinch of salt until they hold firm peaks and fold them gently into the batter, using as few strokes as necessary.

6. Pour olive oil butter over the batter, leaving out the milky sediment at the bottom of the pan.

7. Again using as few strokes as necessary, in order not to deflate the egg whites, scoop in the butter.

8. Spoon the batter into a buttered and floured 9-or 10-inch springform cake pan.

9. Smooth the batter lightly in the pan.

Mangoes with Cinnamon

Preparation time: 5 minutes

Cooking time: 20 minutes

Servings: 4

Ingredients:

- 3 fresh mangoes
- 1 tsp. cinnamon

Directions:

1. You will have two rounded sections of fruit and one flat section with the seed..

2. Slicing down to the skin but not through it, make cuts across the section about every half inch.

3. Turn fruit 90 degrees and make another set of cuts.

4. Hold the mango section in both hands.

5. Using your fingers, push mango skin and turn inside out so the mango flesh will be removed from the cuts made and off the skin.

6. Repeat with other side.

7. Next, peel the middle section.

8. Carefully slice the flesh from the seed.

9. Refrigerate mangoes overnight to chill thoroughly.

10. Place in a dessert dish.

11. Garnish with coconut and sprinkle lightly with cinnamon.

Apricot glaze

Preparation time: 5 minutes

Cooking time: 40 minutes

Servings: 4

Ingredients

- ½ cup apricot pre Servings or jam
- 1 Tbs. sugar

Directions:

1. To make an apricot glaze, just rub the apricot preServings: or jam through a fine sieve, add the sugar, and boil for a few minutes.

2. The mixture will be thick and sticky.

3. Keep it warm over hot water until you need it, and while using it.

4. If it gets too thick to handle, it can be thinned out with a few drops of water.

5. If you don't have a quiche pan or flan ring, a shallow 10-inch pie pan can be used, but I recommend getting a false-bottom quiche pan—they're inexpensive and very useful.

6. The dried beans or rice are used as a weight, to keep the crust from slipping down the sides and puffing up in the middle.

7. Keep the beans or rice in a jar—they can be reused for this purpose indefinitely.

Acai and Banana Smoothie

Preparation time: 10 minutes

Cooking time: 0 minutes

Servings: 3

Ingredients:

- 1 cup of frozen acai

- ¼ cup of coconut milk

- 1 frozen banana

- ½ cup of frozen blueberries

Directions:

1. Put all the ingredients in the juicer or food processor and pulse until liquid.

2. If needed, add some water to make it more liquid depending on the texture that you enjoy.

3. Add a couple of ice cubes

Berries Dip

Preparation time: 15 minutes

Cooking time: 0 minutes

Servings: 6

Ingredients:

- 1 cup blackberries
- 1 cup blueberries
- 1 cup coconut cream
- 1 teaspoon mint, dried
- 1 teaspoon stevia

Directions:

1. In a blender, combine the berries with the cream and the other ingredients, pulse well, divide into small bowls and keep in the fridge for 15 minutes before serving.

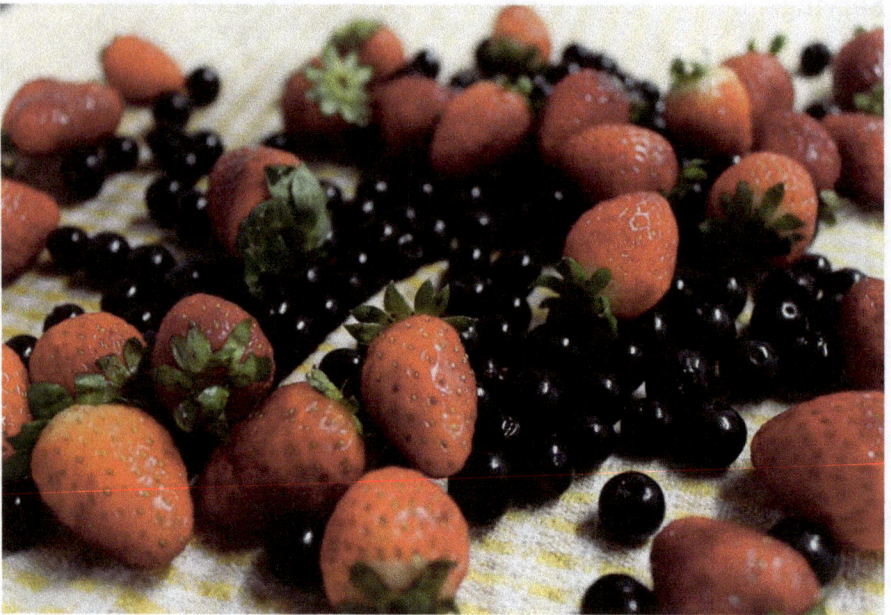

Blueberry and Greens Smoothie

Preparation time: 5 minutes

Cooking time: 0 minutes

Servings: 1

Ingredients:

- ¼ cup coconut milk

- 2 tbsps blueberries

- ½ cup arugula

- 1 tbsp hemp seeds

What you'll need from the store cupboard:

- 2 packets Stevia, or as needed

- 1 ½ cups water

- 3 tbsps coconut oil

Directions

1. Add all ingredients in a blender.

2. Blend until smooth and creamy.

3. Serve and enjoy.

Boysenberry and Greens Shake

Preparation time: 5 minutes

Cooking time: 0 minutes

Servings: 1

Ingredients:

- ¼ cup coconut milk

- 2 tbsps Boysenberry

- 2 packets Stevia, or as needed

- ¼ cup Baby Kale salad mix

- 3 tbsps MCT oil

What you'll need from the store cupboard:

- 1 ½ cups water

Directions

1. Add all ingredients in a blender.

2. Blend until smooth and creamy.

3. Serve and enjoy.

Raspberry-Flavored Chai Smoothie

Preparation time: 5 minutes

Cooking time: 0 minutes

Servings: 1

Ingredients:

- 1 black tea bag

- ¼ tsp ginger

- ¼ tsp cardamom powder

- ¼ cup coconut milk

- 2 tbsps raspberries

What you'll need from the store cupboard:

- 2 packets Stevia or as desired

- 1 ¼ cups boiling water

- ¼ tsp cinnamon

- 3 tbsps MCT oil or coconut oil

Directions

1. Add all ingredients in a blender.

2. Blend until smooth and creamy.

3. Serve and enjoy.

Chai Tea Smoothie

Preparation time: 5 minutes

 Cooking time: 0 minutes

Servings: 1

Ingredients:

- 1 black tea bag

- ¼ tsp ginger

- ¼ tsp cinnamon

- ¼ tsp cardamom powder

- ½ cup coconut milk

What you'll need from the store cupboard:

- 1 cup boiling water

- 2 packets Stevia or as desired

- 3 tbsp MCT oil or coconut oil

Directions

1. Add all ingredients in a blender.

2. Blend until smooth and creamy.

3. Serve and enjoy.

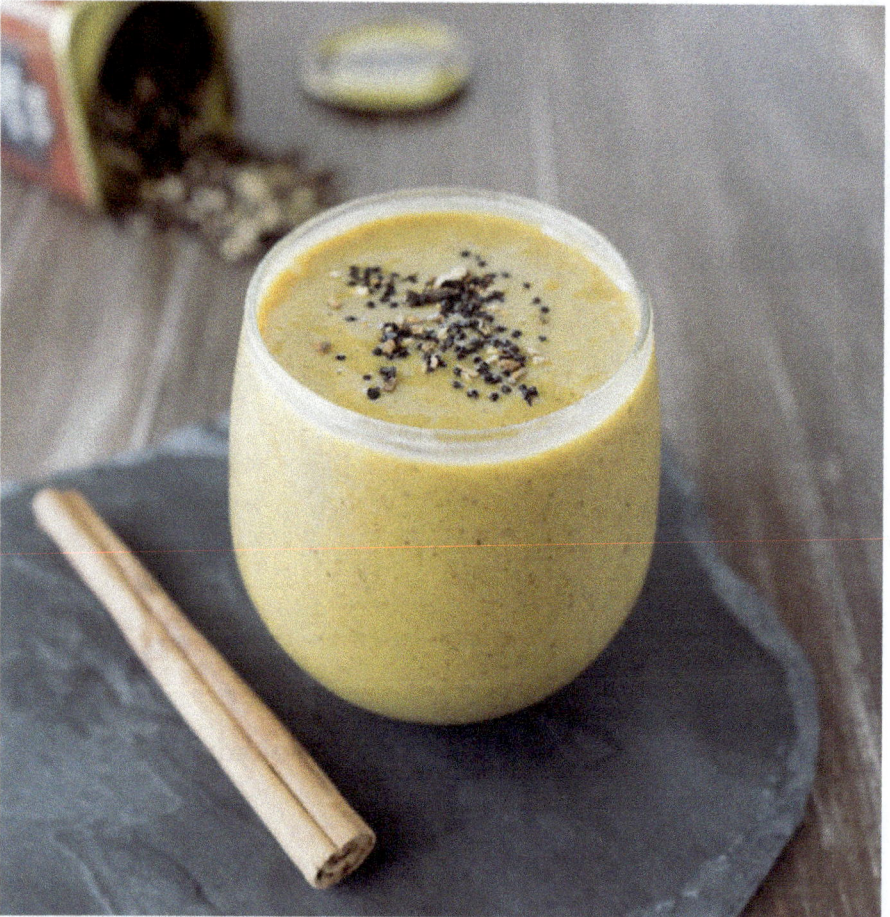

Hemp Green Smoothie

Preparation time: 30 minutes

Cooking time: 0 minutes

Servings: 01

Ingredients:

- ½ cup spinach

- ¼ avocado

- ½ banana, frozen

- 1 tablespoon hemp hearts

- 1 teaspoon chia seeds

- 1 cup almond milk

Directions:

1. Add all ingredients to a blender.

2. Hit the pulse button and blend till it is smooth.

3. Chill well to serve.

Gritty Choco Milk Shake

Preparation time: 5 minutes

Cooking time: 0 minutes

Servings: 1

Ingredients:

- ¼ cup heavy cream
- 1 tbsp chia seeds
- 1 tbsp hemp seeds
- 1 tbsp flaxseed
- 1 tbsp flaxseed oil

What you'll need from the store cupboard:

- 1 ½ cups water
- 1 packet Stevia, or more to taste
- 1 tbsp cocoa powder

- 3 tbsp coconut oil

Directions

1. Add all ingredients in a blender.

2. Blend until smooth and creamy.

3. Serve and enjoy.

High Protein, Green and Fruity Smoothie

Preparation time: 10 minutes

Cooking time: 0 minutes

Servings: 2

Ingredients:

- 1 cup spinach, packed
- ½ small banana, peeled and frozen
- ½ avocado, peeled, pitted, and frozen
- 1 tbsp almond butter
- ¼ cup packed kale, stem discarded, and leaves chopped

What you'll need from the store cupboard:

- 1 cup ice-cold water
- 5 tablespoons MCT oil or coconut oil

Directions

1. Whisk all ingredients in a blender until smooth and creamy.

2. Serve and enjoy.

Nutritiously Green Milk Shake

Preparation time: 10 minutes

Cooking time: 5 minutes

Servings: 1

Ingredients:

- 1 cup coconut cream

- 1 packet Stevia, or more to taste

- 1 tbsp coconut flakes, unsweetened

- 2 cups spring mix salad

- 3 tbsps coconut oil

What you'll need from the store cupboard:

- 1 cup water

Directions

1. Add all ingredients in a mixer.

2. Whisk until smooth and creamy.

3. Serve and enjoy.

Raspberry and Greens Shake

Preparation time: 5 minutes

Cooking time: 0 minutes

Servings: 1

Ingredients:

- ½ cup half and half
- 1 packet Stevia, or more to taste
- 4 raspberries, fresh
- 1 tbsp macadamia oil
- 1 cup Spinach

What you'll need from the store cupboard:

- 1 cup water

Directions

1. Add all ingredients in a mixer.

2. Whisk until smooth and creamy.

3. Serve and enjoy

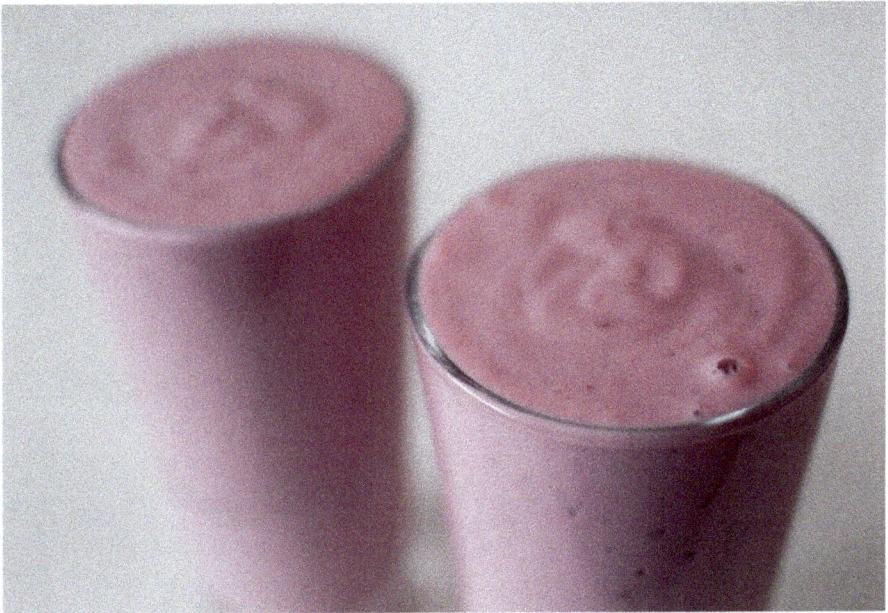

Gritty and Nutty Shake

Preparation time: 5 minutes

Cooking time: 0 minutes

Servings: 1

Ingredients:

- ¼ cup heavy cream, liquid

- 1 tbsp almonds, sliced

- 1 tbsp macadamia nuts, whole

- 1 tbsp flaxseed

- 1 tbsp hemp seed

What you'll need from the store cupboard:

- 1 packet Stevia, or more to taste

- 1 cup water

- ½ tbsp cocoa powder (optional)

- 3 tbsp coconut oil

Directions

1. Add all ingredients in a mixer.

2. Whisk until smooth and creamy.

3. Serve and enjoy

Warm Pomegranate Punch

Servings: 10

Preparation time: 2 hours and 15 minutes

Ingredients:

- 3 cinnamon sticks, each about 3 inches long

- 12 whole cloves

- 1/2 cup of coconut sugar

- 1/3 cup of lemon juice

- 32 fluid ounce of pomegranate juice

- 32 fluid ounce of apple juice, unsweetened

- 16 fluid ounce of brewed tea

Directions:

1. Using a 4-quart slow cooker, pour the lemon juice, pomegranate, juice apple juice, tea, and then sugar.

2. Wrap the whole cloves and cinnamon stick in a cheese cloth, tie its corners with a string, and immerse it in the liquid present in the slow cooker.

3. Then cover it with the lid, plug in the slow cooker and let it cook at the low heat setting for 3 hours or until it is heated thoroughly.

4. When done, discard the cheesecloth bag and serve it hot or cold.

Apple and Cucumber Juice

Preparation time: 10 minutes

Cooking time: 0 minutes

Servings: 2

Ingredients:

- 3 apples
- 1 cucumber
- 2 celery stick
- 1 cup of vegetable milk Cinnamon, to taste
- Chia seeds (optional)

Directions:

1. Wash the apple, cucumber, and celery stick thoroughly.
2. Chop the three in small pieces.

3. Add them to the juicer or food processor along with the vegetable milk you chose and the cinnamon.

4. If you wish to, top with some chia seeds and add a couple of ice cubes.

Minty-Coco and Greens Shake

Preparation time: 5 minutes

Cooking time: 0 minutes

Servings: 1

Ingredients:

- ½ cup coconut milk

- 2 peppermint leaves

- 2 packets Stevia, or as needed

- 1 cup 50/50 salad mix

- 1 tbsp coconut oil

What you'll need from the store cupboard:

- 1 ½ cups water

Directions

1. Add all ingredients in a blender.

2. Blend until smooth and creamy.

3. Serve and enjoy.

Turmeric Lassi

Preparation time: 5 minutes

Cooking time: 0 minute

Servings: 2

Ingredients:

- 1 teaspoon grated ginger

- 1/8 teaspoon ground black pepper

- 1 teaspoon turmeric powder

- 1/8 teaspoon cayenne

- 1 tablespoon coconut sugar

- 1/8 teaspoon salt

- 1 cup vegan yogurt

- 1 cup almond milk

Directions:

1. Place all the ingredients in the order in a food processor or blender and then pulse for 2 to 3 minutes at high speed until smooth.

2. Pour the lassi into two glasses and then serve.

Saffron Pistachio Beverage

Preparation time: 5 minutes

Cooking time: 0 minute

Servings: 2

Ingredients:

- 8 strands of saffron

- 1 tablespoon cashews

- 1/4 teaspoon ground ginger

- 2 tablespoons pistachio

- 1/8 teaspoon cloves

- 1/4 teaspoon ground black pepper

- 1/4 teaspoon cardamom powder

- 3 tablespoons coconut sugar

- 1/4 teaspoon cinnamon

- 1/8 teaspoon fennel seeds

- 1/4 teaspoon poppy seeds

Directions:

1. Place all the ingredients in the order in a food processor or blender and then pulse for 2 to 3 minutes at high speed until smooth.

2. Pour the smoothie into two glasses and then serve.

Pumpkin Spice Frappuccino

Preparation time: 5 minutes

Cooking time: 0 minute

Servings: 2

Ingredients:

- ½ teaspoon ground ginger 1/8 teaspoon allspice

- ½ teaspoon ground cinnamon

- 2 tablespoons coconut sugar

- 1/8 teaspoon nutmeg

- ¼ teaspoon ground cloves

- 1 teaspoon vanilla extract, unsweetened

- 2 teaspoons instant coffee

- 2 cups almond milk, unsweetened

- 1 cup of ice cubes

Directions:

1. Place all the ingredients in the order in a food processor or blender and then pulse for 2 to 3 minutes at high speed until smooth.

2. Pour the Frappuccino into two glasses and then serve.

Strawberry and Hemp Smoothie

Preparation time: 5 minutes

Cooking time: 0 minute

Servings: 2

Ingredients:

- 3 cups fresh strawberries

- 2 tablespoons hemp seeds

- 1/2 teaspoon vanilla extract, unsweetened

- 1/8 teaspoon sea salt

- 2 tablespoons maple syrup

- 1 cup vegan yogurt

- 1 cup almond milk, unsweetened

- 1 cup of ice cubes

- 2 tablespoons hemp protein

Directions:

1. Place all the ingredients in the order in a food processor or blender, except for protein powder, and then pulse for 2 to 3 minutes at high speed until smooth.

2. Pour the smoothie into two glasses and then serve.

Mango Lassi

Preparation time: 5 minutes

Cooking time: 0 minute

Servings: 2

Ingredients:

- 1 ¼ cup mango pulp
- 1 tablespoon coconut sugar
- 1/8 teaspoon salt
- 1/2 teaspoon lemon juice
- 1/4 cup almond milk, unsweetened
- 1/4 cup chilled water
- 1 cup cashew yogurt

Directions:

1. Place all the ingredients in the order in a food processor or blender and then pulse for 2 to 3 minutes at high speed until smooth.

2. Pour the lassi into two glasses and then serve.

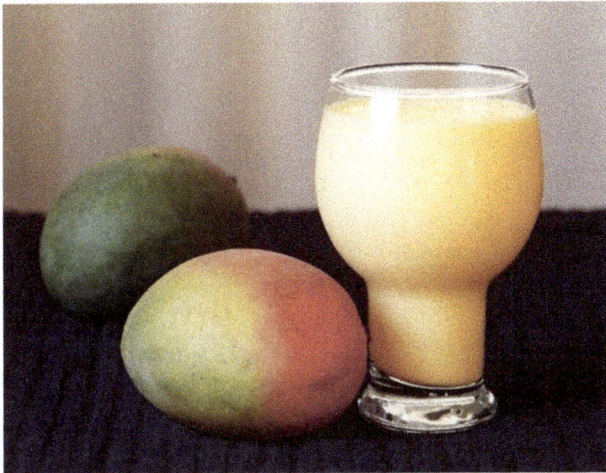

Chard, Lettuce and Ginger Smoothie

Preparation time: 5 minutes

Cooking time: 0 minute

Servings: 2

Ingredients:

- 10 Chard leaves, chopped 1-inch piece of ginger, chopped
- 10 lettuce leaves, chopped
- ½ teaspoon black salt
- 2 pear, chopped
- 2 teaspoons coconut sugar
- ¼ teaspoon ground black pepper
- ¼ teaspoon salt
- 2 tablespoons lemon juice

- 2 cups of water

Directions:

1. Place all the ingredients in the order in a food processor or blender and then pulse for 2 to 3 minutes at high speed until smooth.

2. Pour the smoothie into two glasses and then serve.

Berry and Yogurt Smoothie

Preparation time: 5 minutes

Cooking time: 0 minute

Servings: 2

Ingredients:

- 2 small bananas

- 3 cups frozen mixed berries

- 1 ½ cup cashew yogurt

- 1/2 teaspoon vanilla extract, unsweetened

- 1/2 cup almond milk, unsweetened

Directions:

1. Place all the ingredients in the order in a food processor or blender and then pulse for 2 to 3 minutes at high speed until smooth.

2. Pour the smoothie into two glasses and then serve.

Strawberry and Chocolate Milkshake

Preparation time: 5 minutes

Cooking time: 0 minute

Servings: 2

Ingredients:

- 2 cups frozen strawberries
- 3 tablespoons cocoa powder
- 1 scoop protein powder
- 2 tablespoons maple syrup
- 1 teaspoon vanilla extract, unsweetened
- 2 cups almond milk, unsweetened

Directions:

1. Place all the ingredients in the order in a food processor or blender and then pulse for 2 to 3 minutes at high speed until smooth.

2. Pour the smoothie into two glasses and then serve.

Mango, Pineapple and Banana Smoothie

Preparation time: 5 minutes

Cooking time: 0 minute

Servings: 2

Ingredients:

- 2 cups pineapple chunks

- 2 frozen bananas

- 2 medium mangoes, destoned, cut into chunks

- 1 cup almond milk, unsweetened

- Chia seeds as needed for garnishing

Directions:

1. Place all the ingredients in the order in a food processor or blender and then pulse for 2 to 3 minutes at high speed until smooth.

2. Pour the smoothie into two glasses and then serve.

Spiced Buttermilk

Preparation time: 5 minutes

Cooking time: 0 minute

Servings: 2

Ingredients:

- 3/4 teaspoon ground cumin

- 1/4 teaspoon sea salt

- 1/8 teaspoon ground black pepper

- 2 mint leaves

- 1/8 teaspoon lemon juice

- ¼ cup cilantro leaves

- 1 cup of chilled water

- 1 cup vegan yogurt, unsweetened

- Ice as needed

Directions:

1. Place all the ingredients in the order in a food processor or blender, except for cilantro and ¼ teaspoon cumin, and then pulse for 2 to 3 minutes at high speed until smooth.

2. Pour the milk into glasses, top with cilantro and cumin, and then serve.

Brownie Batter Orange Chia Shake

Preparation time: 5 minutes

Cooking time: 0 minute

Servings: 2

Ingredients:

- 2 tablespoons cocoa powder
- 3 tablespoons chia seeds
- ¼ teaspoon salt
- 4 tablespoons chocolate chips
- 4 teaspoons coconut sugar
- ½ teaspoon orange zest
- ½ teaspoon vanilla extract, unsweetened
- 2 cup almond milk

Directions:

1. Place all the ingredients in the order in a food processor or blender and then pulse for 2 to 3 minutes at high speed until smooth.

2. Pour the smoothie into two glasses and then serve.

Mexican Hot Chocolate Mix

Preparation time: 5 minutes

Cooking time: 0 minute

Servings: 2

Ingredients:

For the Hot Chocolate Mix:

- 1/3 cup chopped dark chocolate

- 1/8 teaspoon cayenne

- 1/8 teaspoon salt

- 1/2 teaspoon cinnamon

- 1/4 cup coconut sugar

- 1 teaspoon cornstarch

- 3 tablespoons cocoa powder

- 1/2 teaspoon vanilla extract, unsweetened

For Serving:

- 2 cups milk, warmed

Directions:

1. Place all the ingredients of hot chocolate mix in the order in a food processor or blender and then pulse for 2 to 3 minutes at high speed until ground.

2. Stir 2 tablespoons of the chocolate mix into a glass of milk until combined and then serve.

Cookie Dough Milkshake

Preparation time: 5 minutes

Cooking time: 0 minute

Servings: 2

Ingredients:

- 2 tablespoons cookie dough

- 5 dates, pitted

- 2 teaspoons chocolate chips

- 1/2 teaspoon vanilla extract, unsweetened

- 1/2 cup almond milk, unsweetened

- 1 ½ cup almond milk ice cubes

Directions:

1. Place all the ingredients in the order in a food processor or blender and then pulse for 2 to 3 minutes at high speed until smooth.

2. Pour the milkshake into two glasses and then serve with some cookie dough balls.

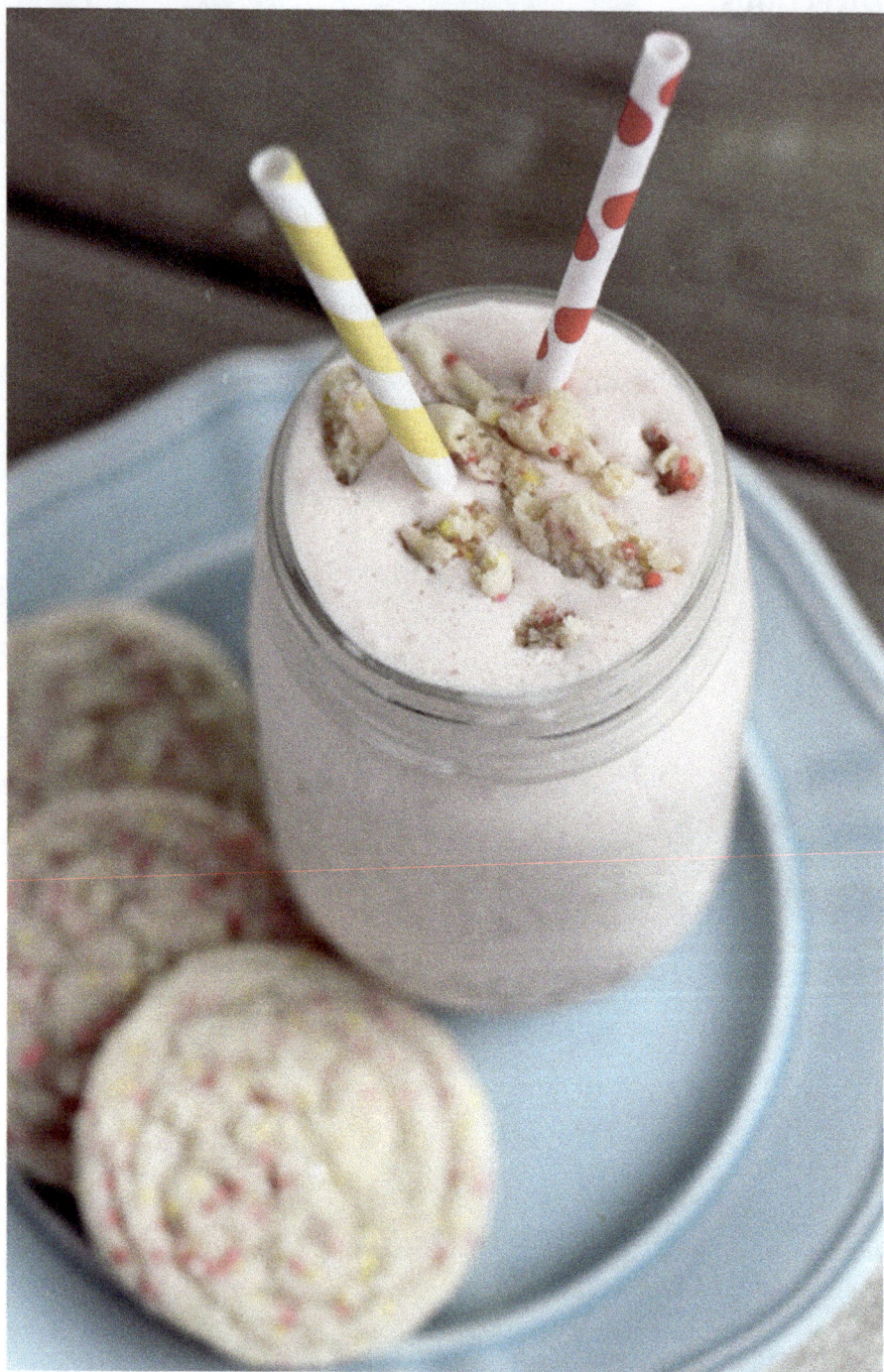

www.ingramcontent.com/pod-product-compliance
Lightning Source LLC
Chambersburg PA
CBHW050750030426
42336CB00012B/1746